The Healthy Ketogenic Cookbook for Beginners

Delicious Ketogenic Recipes to Boost Your Diet and Manage Your Weight

I0134873

Lauren Loose

© Copyright 2021 - All rights reserved.

The content contained within this book may not be reproduced, duplicated or transmitted without direct written permission from the author or the publisher.

Under no circumstances will any blame or legal responsibility be held against the publisher, or author, for any damages, reparation, or monetary loss due to the information contained within this book. Either directly or indirectly.

Legal Notice:

This book is copyright protected. This book is only for personal use. You cannot amend, distribute, sell, use, quote or paraphrase any part, or the content within this book, without the consent of the author or publisher.

Disclaimer Notice:

Please note the information contained within this document is for educational and entertainment purposes only. All effort has been executed to present accurate, up to date, and reliable, complete information. No warranties of any kind are declared or implied. Readers acknowledge that the author is not engaging in the rendering of legal, financial, medical or professional advice. The content within this book has been derived from various sources. Please consult a licensed professional before attempting any techniques outlined in this book.

By reading this document, the reader agrees that under no circumstances is the author responsible for any losses, direct or indirect, which are incurred as a result of the use of information contained within this document, including, but not limited to, — errors, omissions, or inaccuracies.

Contents

Instant Pot Chili Verde

Preparation Time: 10 minutes

Cooking Time: 40 minutes

Servings: 4

Ingredient:

- 2 lbs. boneless skinless chicken thighs
- 12 oz tomatillos, husked and quartered
- 8 oz poblano peppers stemmed, seeded, and chopped
- 4 oz jalapeño peppers stemmed, seeded, and chopped
- 4 oz onions chopped
- 1/4 cup water
- 1 1/2 tsp salt
- 2 tsp ground cumin
- 5 cloves garlic
- ¼ oz chopped cilantro leaves (for finishing)
- 1 tbsp fresh lime juice (for finishing)

Directions:

1. Put the poblanos, jalapenos, onions, and tomatillos in a pressure cooker. Add the water and sprinkle the cumin, salt, and garlic on top. Put the chicken inside and seal the lid. Turn the pressure on high for 15 minutes.

2. Release the pressure and uncover the lid. Put the chicken on a cutting board and cut it into small pieces. Set it aside. Add cilantro and lime juice to the pressure cooker. Choose the sauté mode on the pressure cooker.
3. Put the chicken back to the mixture and boil for the next 10 minutes to cause the chicken sauce to thicken. Stir it occasionally. Serve and garnish with more cilantro if you want.

Nutrition:

310 calories

15g total fat

10g total carbohydrates

Ingredient Ketogenic Salad

Preparation Time: 15 minutes

Cooking Time: 0 minute

Servings: 2

Ingredient:

- 2 boneless chicken breasts with skin
- 1 large avocado, sliced
- 3 slices of bacon
- 4 cups mixed leafy greens of choice
- 2 tbsp. dairy-free ranch dressing
- Salt and pepper to taste
- Duck fat for greasing

Directions:

1. Start by preheating the oven to 200 degrees Celsius or 400 degrees Fahrenheit. Season the chicken with salt and pepper. Grab a skillet and grease it with duck fat before cooking the chicken on the hot pan. Keep the heat on high until you get a golden-brown skin surface. This should take around 5 minutes per side.

2. Once done, you can cook the chicken in the oven for 10 to 15 minutes. You can also put the bacon in with the chicken to save on the

cooking time. You can also fry it in a pan, depending your personal preferences.

3. After cooking, let the chicken rest for a few minutes. Slice the avocado and the cooked chicken. Start assembling your salad, adding together the leafy greens, crispy bacon, sliced chicken, and avocado.

4. Use 2 tablespoons of ranch dressing. Mix together until all ingredients are thoroughly coated. Enjoy!

Nutrition:

3.1g carbs

38.7g protein

43.8g fat

Vegetarian Ketogenic Cobb

Preparation Time: 10 minutes

Cooking Time: 0 minute

Servings: 3

Ingredient:

- 3 large hard-boiled eggs, sliced
- 4 ounces cheddar cheese, cubed
- 2 tbsp. sour cream
- 2 tbsp. mayonnaise
- ½ tsp. garlic powder
- ½ tsp. onion powder
- 1 tsp. dried parsley
- 1 tbsp. milk
- 1 tbsp. Dijon mustard
- 3 cups romaine lettuce, torn
- 1 cup cucumber, diced
- ½ cup cherry tomatoes, halved

Directions:

1. The dressing is a combination of the source cream, mayonnaise, and dried herbs. Mix them well together until full combined. Add one tablespoon of milk into the mix until you get the thickness you want.

2. Layer in the salad, adding all the ingredients that's not part of the dressing recipe. Put the mustard on the center of the salad. Drizzle with your dressing and enjoy! Each serving should have just 2 tablespoons of dressing.

Nutrition:

330 calories

26.32g fat

16.82g protein

Quinoa Salad

Preparation Time: 5 minutes

Cooking Time: 5 minutes

Serving: 4

Ingredients:

- 1 red bell pepper
- 1 cup water
- ¾ cup dry quinoa
- 1 carrot
- 1 bunch green onions
- 1 jalapeno
- 1 batch peanut sauce
- 1 boiled chicken breast
- ¼ cup dry roasted peanuts

Directions:

1. Cook quinoa according to the instructions. In a bowl add all ingredients and mix well. Serve with dressing.

Nutrition:

296 calories

12 g fat

900 mg sodium.

Yellow-Beet Salad

Preparation Time: 5 minutes

Cooking Time: 5 minutes

Serving: 4

Ingredients:

- 10 oz. cooked yellow beets
- 3 oz. anchovies
- ¼ red onion
- 1 cup mayonnaise
- 2 endive lettuce

Directions:

1. In a bowl add all ingredients and mix well. Serve with dressing

Nutrition:

180 Calories

10g Sugar

380mg Sodium

14g Fat

Ketogenic Caesar Salad

Preparation Time: 5 minutes

Cooking Time: 5 minutes

Serving: 4

Ingredients:

- 8 oz. chicken breasts
- 1 tablespoon olive oil
- salt
- 2 oz. bacon
- 6 oz. romaine lettuce
- 1 oz. parmesan cheese

Dressing

- ¼ cup mayonnaise
- 1 tablespoon mustard
- ¼ lemon
- 1 tablespoon parmesan cheese
- 1 tablespoon anchovies
- 1 garlic clove

Directions:

1. In a bowl add all ingredients and mix well. Serve with dressing

Nutrition:

418 Calories

3g Carbohydrates

20g Protein

35g Fat

Ketogenic Salad Niçoise

Preparation Time: 5 minutes

Cooking Time: 5 minutes

Serving: 4

Ingredients:

- 2 eggs
- 2 oz. celery root
- 4 oz. green beans
- 2 tablespoons olive oil
- 2 garlic cloves
- 4 oz. romaine lettuce
- 2 oz. cherry tomatoes
- ¼ red onion
- 1 can tuna
- 2 oz. olives

Dressing

- 2 tablespoons capers
- ¼ oz. anchovies
- ½ cup olive oil
- ½ cup mayonnaise
- ¼ lemon
- 1 tablespoon parsley

Directions:

1. In a bowl sauté peppers in coconut oil. In a bowl add all ingredients and mix well. Serve with dressing

Nutrition:

6g Fiber

85g Fat

34g Protein

957 Calories

Greek Salad

Preparation Time: 5 minutes

Cooking Time: 5 minutes

Serving: 4

Ingredients:

- 2 ripe tomatoes
- ¼ cucumber
- ¼ red onion
- ¼ green bell pepper
- 6 oz. feta cheese
- 8 black Greek olives
- 5 tablespoons olive oil
- ¼ tablespoon red wine vinegar
- 2 tsp oregano

Directions:

1. In a bowl add all ingredients and mix well. Serve with dressing

Nutrition:

142 Calories

10g Carbs

9g Fat

9g Protein

Ketogenic Chicken Salad

Preparation Time: 5 minutes

Cooking Time: 5 minutes

Serving: 4

Ingredients:

- 1 lb. boneless chicken thighs
- 1 oz. butter
- ¼ lb. bacon
- 3 oz. cherry tomatoes
- 8 oz. romaine lettuce

Dressing

- ½ cup mayonnaise
- ¼ tablespoon garlic powder

Directions:

1. In a bowl add all ingredients and mix well. Serve with dressing

Nutrition:

175 Calories

12g Fat

16g Protein

Ketogenic Cobb Salad

Preparation Time: 5 minutes

Cooking Time: 5 minutes

Serving: 4

Ingredients:

- 2 hard-boiled eggs
- 4 oz. bacon
- ¼ rotisserie chicken
- 3 oz. blue cheese
- 1 tomato
- 4 oz. iceberg lettuce
- 1 tablespoon chives

Ranch dressing

- 2 tablespoons mayonnaise
- 1 tablespoon ranch seasoning
- 1 tablespoon water

Directions:

1. In a bowl add all ingredients and mix well. Serve with dressing

Nutrition:

726 Calories

14g Carbohydrates

17g Protein

67g Fat

Tomato Salad

Preparation Time: 5 minutes

Cooking Time: 5 minutes

Serving: 4

Ingredients:

- 1 bunch spinach
- 6-pieces bacon
- 2 red beets
- 2 tomatoes
- 1 cup walnuts
- ½ tsp salt
- 1 tsp black pepper
- 5 tablespoons garlic infused oil

Directions:

1. In a bowl add all ingredients and mix well. Serve with dressing

Nutrition:

92 Calories

9g Fat

7g Carbohydrates

1g Protein

Coleslaw

Preparation Time: 5 minutes

Cooking Time: 5 minutes

Serving: 4

Ingredients:

- 1 carrot
- ½ red cabbage
- 1 handful parsley
- 2 scallions
- 2 tablespoon mayonnaise
- salt

Directions:

1. In a bowl add all ingredients and mix well. Serve with dressing

Nutrition:

180 Calories

3g Carbs

16g Fat:

3g Protein

Salmon and Cherry

Tomatoes Salad

Preparation Time: 5 minutes

Cooking Time: 5 minutes

Serving: 4

Ingredients:

3 oz. smoked salmon

½ oz. leafy greens

½ oz. cherry tomatoes

½ oz. red bell peppers

½ oz. cucumber

¼ scallion

3 tablespoons mayonnaise

Directions:

In a bowl add all ingredients and mix well. Serve with dressing

Nutrition:

554 Calories

29.4g Total Fat

8.1g Saturated Fat

4.3g Polyunsaturated Fat

11. Antipasto Salad

Preparation Time: 5 minutes

Cooking Time: 5 minutes

Serving: 4

Ingredients:

- 12 oz. romaine lettuce
- 3 tablespoon parsley
- 4 oz. mozzarella cheese
- 3 oz. ham
- 3 oz. salami
- 4 oz. canned artichokes
- 2 oz. roasted red peppers
- 1 oz. sun-dried tomatoes
- 2 tablespoons olives
- ½ cup basil
- 1 red chili pepper
- ¼ tablespoon salt

Directions:

1. In a bowl add all ingredients and mix well. Serve with dressing

Nutrition:

11g Total Fat

9g Total Carbohydrate

3g Dietary Fiber

19g Protein

Ketogenic Avocado and

Bacon Salad

Preparation Time: 5 minutes

Cooking Time: 5 minutes

Serving: 4

Ingredients:

- 8 oz. cheese
- 6 oz. bacon
- 2 avocados
- 3 oz. walnuts
- 3 oz. arugula lettuce

Dressing

- ¼ lemon
- ¼ cup mayonnaise
- ¼ cup olive oil
- 1 tablespoon heavy cream

Directions:

1. In a bowl add all ingredients and mix well. Serve with dressing

Nutrition:

9g Fiber

123g Fat

27g Protein

1251 Calories

Pastrami Salad with Croutons

Preparation Time: 5 minutes

Cooking Time: 15 minutes

Serving: 4

Ingredients:

- 1 cup mayonnaise
- 1 tablespoon mustard
- 1 shallot
- 1 dill pickle
- 6 oz. lettuce
- 9 oz. pastrami
- 4 eggs
- 6 low-carb parmesan croutons

Directions:

1. In a bowl add all ingredients and mix well. Serve with dressing.

Nutrition:

456.0 Calories

39.6 g Total Fat

11.8 g Total Carbohydrate

Ketogenic Hoagie Bowl

Preparation Time: 5 minutes

Cooking Time: 5 minutes

Serving: 4

Ingredients:

- 10 oz. roast turkey
- 10 oz. salami
- 10 oz. smoked ham
- 10 oz. provolone cheese
- 6 oz. cheese
- 2 cups lettuce
- 1 cup tomatoes
- ¼ cup cucumber
- ¼ cup red onion

Dressing

- ¼ cup mayonnaise
- ½ cup red wine vinegar
- 1 tablespoon olive oil
- 1 tsp dried basil
- ¼ tsp. Italian seasoning
- ¼ tsp. dried oregano

Directions:

1. In a bowl add all ingredients and mix well. Serve with dressing

Nutrition:

1g Fiber

35g Fat

21g Protein

421 Calories

Cucumber Salad

Preparation Time: 5 minutes

Cooking Time: 5 minutes

Serving: 4

Ingredients:

- 1 cucumber
- 1 cup cherry tomatoes
- juice of ½ lime
- ¼ cup olive oil
- 1 tsp oregano
- ¼ tsp. salt

Directions:

1. In a bowl add all ingredients and mix well. Serve with dressing

Nutrition:

19 Calories

5g Carbs

0g Fat

1g Protein

Artichoke Shrimp Pasta Salad

Preparation Time: 10 minutes

Cooking Time: 10 minutes

Servings: 12

Ingredients:

- 1 package (16 oz.) bow tie pasta
- 2 lbs. peeled and deveined cooked shrimp (31-40 per lb.)
- 2 cans (7-1/2 oz. each) marinated quartered artichoke hearts, drained
- 2 cans (2-1/4 oz. each) sliced ripe olives, drained
- 2 cups (8 oz.) crumbled feta cheese
- 8 green onions, sliced
- 1/2 cup chopped fresh parsley
- 1/4 cup chopped fresh basil

Dressing:

- 1/2 cup white wine vinegar
- 1/2 cup olive oil
- 1/4 cup lemon juice
- 2 tbsps. chopped fresh basil
- 2 tsps. Dijon mustard
- Fresh ground pepper, optional

Directions:

1. Follow the cooking instructions on the package to cook the pasta for it to cook through, but is still firm to the bite. Drain well and rinse with cold water and drain again. Mix basil, parsley, green onions, cheese, olives, artichokes, shrimp and pasta together in a large bowl.
2. To make the dressing, whisk pepper (optional), mustard, basil, lemon juice, oil and vinegar in a small bowl. Toss the pasta mixture with the dressing to coat. Cover and place in the fridge 2 hours prior to serving.

Nutrition:

312 Calories

38.4g Carbohydrates

17.6g Protein

9.4g Fat

6.6g Fiber

Artichoke Tomato Salad

Preparation Time: 12 minutes

Cooking Time: 8 minutes

Servings: 8

Ingredients:

- 5 large tomatoes (about 2 lbs.), cut into wedges
- 1/4 tsp. salt
- 1/4 tsp. pepper
- 1 jar (7-1/2 oz.) marinated quartered artichoke hearts, drained
- 1 can (2-1/4 oz.) sliced ripe olives, drained
- 2 tbsps. minced fresh parsley
- 2 tbsps. white wine vinegar
- 2 garlic cloves, minced

Directions:

1. Lay tomato wedges on a large platter; use salt and pepper to sprinkle. Toss remaining ingredients in a small bowl; transfer the mixture over tomatoes.

Nutrition:

74 calories

7g Total Carbohydrate

5g Total Fat

2g Fiber

Asparagus-Fennel Pasta Salad

Preparation Time: 15 minutes

Cooking Time: 10 minutes

Servings: 14

Ingredients:

- 1 lb. fresh asparagus, trimmed and cut into 3/4-inch pieces
- 2 medium onions, halved and thinly sliced
- 1 small fennel bulb, sliced
- 2 tbsps. olive oil
- 8 oz. uncooked penne pasta
- 4 medium tomatoes, seeded and diced
- 12 pitted Greek olives, sliced
- 1 cup minced fresh parsley

Vinaigrette:

- 1/4 cup olive oil
- 1/4 cup lemon juice
- 2 garlic cloves, minced
- 1/2 tsp. Dijon mustard
- 1/2 tsp. salt
- 1/4 tsp. pepper
- 1 cup (4 oz.) crumbled feta cheese

Directions:

1. Place fennel, onions, and asparagus in a 15x10x1-inch baking pan. Drizzle oil over the vegetables and stir until evenly coated. Bake for 20 to 25 minutes at 400 degrees or until crisp-tender and lightly brown, stirring sometimes.

2. In the meantime, cook pasta as directed on the package. Drain off water and transfer pasta into a large serving bowl. Add roasted vegetables, parsley, olives, and tomatoes.

3. Combine pepper, salt, mustard, garlic, lemon juice, and oil in a small bowl, stir properly. Pour dressing over salad and toss until evenly coated. Top with feta cheese before serving.

Nutrition:

167 calories

19g Total Carbohydrate

8g Total Fat

3g Fiber

5g Protein

Balsamic Cucumber Salad

Preparation Time: 10 minutes

Cooking Time: 5 minutes

Servings: 6

Ingredients:

- 1 large English cucumber, halved and sliced
- 2 cups grape tomatoes, halved
- 1 medium red onion, halved and thinly sliced
- 1/2 cup balsamic vinaigrette
- 3/4 cup crumbled reduced-fat feta cheese

Directions:

1. Mix onion, tomatoes, and cucumber in a big bowl. Add in vinaigrette and mix to coat. Put in the fridge, cover it until serving. Mix in cheese before eating. Use a slotted spoon to eat.

Nutrition:

90 calories

9g Total Carbohydrate

5g Total Fat

1g Fiber

4g Protein

Beet and Arugula Salad

Preparation Time: 15 minutes

Cooking Time: 5 minutes

Servings: 4

Ingredients:

- 2 lbs. beets, trimmed
- 4 small garlic cloves, minced
- 1 1/2 tsps. salt
- 5 tbsps. fresh lemon juice, or to taste
- 1/2 lb. arugula
- 1 (8 oz.) package feta cheese, thinly sliced
- 16 pitted kalamata olives
- 1/4 cup olive oil, divided

Directions:

1. Put beets into a big saucepan and fill in enough water so that the water level is 1 inch higher than the beets. Boil the water then lower the heat to medium-low, use a lid to cover and let simmer for about 15 minutes till you are able to use a fork to pierce the beets easily. Drain and allow them to cool.

2. Peel the beets, chop into 1/4-inch thick pieces, and then slice in half. Put sliced beets into a bowl.

3. In a small bowl, use a spoon to smash garlic with salt to make sure the mixture becomes a paste. Pour lemon juice into the garlic paste then stir. Keep about a tbsp. of lemon dressing in a small bowl. For the remaining lemon dressing, pour over the beets and stir to make sure the beets are coated with dressing.

4. Distribute arugula among 4 plates, add olives, feta cheese, beets on top of each plate; pour drizzles of the lemon dressing you set aside before and olive oil on top of the salad.

Nutrition:

432 calories

30.1g Total Carbohydrate

51mg Cholesterol

30.3g Total Fat

13.7g Protein

Crunchy Strawberry Salad

Preparation time: 10 minutes

Cooking time: 0 minutes

Servings: 5

Ingredients:

- 0.6 lb. romaine lettuce leaves, roughly torn
- 0.6 lb. strawberries, sliced
- 0.2 lb. nuts of choice

Directions:

1. In a large mixing bowl add strawberry slices, lettuce, and nuts; toss to combine.
2. Add to a serving bowl.

Nutrition:

94 Calories

3g Fat

22g Carbohydrates

11g Protein

Lunch Caesar Salad

Preparation Time: 15 minutes

Cooking time: 10 minutes

Servings: 2

Ingredients:

- 1 avocado, pitted
- 1 chicken breast, grilled and shredded
- 1 cup bacon, cooked and crumbled
- 3 tbsp creamy Caesar dressing
- Salt and ground black pepper to taste

Directions:

1. Peel and slice avocado. In medium bowl, combine bacon, chicken breast and avocado.
2. Add creamy Cesar dressing, stir well. Season with salt and pepper, stir. Serve.

Nutrition:

329 Calories

2.99g Carbs

22.9g Fat

17.8g Protein

Asian Side Salad

Preparation Time: 35 minutes

Cooking Time: 12 minutes

Servings: 4

Ingredients:

- 1 green onion
- 1 cucumber
- 2 tbsp coconut oil
- 1 packet Asian noodles, cooked
- ¼ tsp red pepper flakes
- 1 tbsp sesame oil
- 1 tbsp balsamic vinegar
- 1 tsp sesame seeds
- Salt and ground black pepper to taste

Directions:

1. Chop onion. Slice cucumber thin. Preheat pan with oil on medium high heat. Add cooked noodles and close lid.
2. Fry noodles for 5 minutes until crispy. Transfer noodles to paper towels and drain grease.
3. Combine cucumber, pepper flakes, green onion, sesame oil, vinegar, sesame seeds, pepper, salt and noodles. Mix well. Put in refrigerator at least for 20-30 minutes. Serve.

Nutrition:

397 Calories

3.97g Carbs

33.7g Fat

1.98g Protein

Ketogenic Egg Salad

Preparation Time: 15 minutes

Cooking Time: 10 minutes

Servings: 4

Ingredients:

- 6 oz ham, chopped
- 5 eggs, boiled and chopped
- 1 tsp garlic, minced
- ½ tsp basil
- 1 tsp oregano
- 1 tbsp apple cider vinegar
- 1 tsp kosher salt
- ½ cup cream cheese

Directions:

1. In medium bowl, combine chopped ham with chopped eggs, stir. In another bowl, mix together garlic, basil, oregano, vinegar, and salt. Stir the mixture till you get homogeneous consistency.
2. Whisk together spice mixture and cream cheese. Add cream cheese sauce to egg mixture and stir gently. Serve.

Nutrition:

341 Calories

26g Fat

22.1g Protein

Cobb Salad

Preparation Time: 20 minutes

Cooking Time: 27 minutes

Servings: 1

Ingredients:

- 1 tbsp olive oil
- 4 oz chicken breast
- 2 strips bacon
- 1 cup spinach, chopped roughly
- 1 large hard-boiled egg, peeled and chopped
- ¼ avocado, peeled and chopped
- ½ tsp white vinegar

Directions:

1. Heat up pan on medium heat and add oil. Add chicken breast and bacon, cook until get desired crispiness.
2. Add spinach and egg, stir. Add avocado and mix well. Sprinkle with white vinegar and stir.
3. Serve.

Nutrition:

589Calories

47.8g Fat

42g Protein

Bacon and Zucchini

Noodles Salad

Preparation Time: 15 minutes

Cooking Time: 10 minutes

Servings: 3

Ingredients:

- 32 oz zucchini noodles
- 1 cup baby spinach
- 1/3 cup blue cheese, crumbled
- ½ cup bacon, cooked and crumbled
- 1/3 cup blue cheese dressing
- Ground black pepper to taste

Directions:

1. Combine zucchini noodles, spinach, blue cheese, and bacon, stir carefully.
2. Add black pepper and cheese dressing, toss to coat. Serve.

Nutrition:

198 Calories

13.9g Fat

9.95g Protein

Chicken Salad

Preparation Time: 15 minutes

Cooking Time: 10 minutes

Servings: 3

Ingredients:

- 1 celery stalk
- 2 tbsp fresh parsley
- 1 green onion
- 5 oz chicken breast, roasted and chopped
- 1 egg, hard-boiled, peeled and chopped
- Salt and ground black pepper to taste
- ½ tsp garlic powder
- 1/3 cup mayonnaise
- 1 tsp mustard
- ½ tbsp dill relish

Directions:

1. Wash and chop celery, parsley and onion. Place celery, onion and parsley in blender or food processor and blend well. Remove this mass from food processor and set aside.

2. Place chicken in food processor and pulse well. Add chicken to onion mixture and stir. Add egg, pepper and salt, stir gently. Add garlic powder,

mayonnaise, and mustard and dill relish, toss
to coat.

3. Serve.

Nutrition:

279 Calories

22.9g Fat

11.9g Protein

Asparagus Salad

Preparation Time: 20 minutes

Cooking Time: 5 minutes

Servings: 5

Ingredients:

- 2 lbs. asparagus, cooked and halved
- 1 tbsp butter, melted
- ½ tsp garlic powder
- 1 tsp sesame seeds
- 1 tbsp coconut oil
- 1 tbsp apple cider vinegar
- 1 tsp dried basil
- 1 tsp salt
- 4 oz Parmesan cheese, grated

Directions:

1. In bowl, combine asparagus, butter and garlic powder. Stir well. Add sesame seeds, coconut oil, vinegar, basil and salt. Mix well.
2. Set salad aside to marinate. Serve salad with grated Parmesan cheese.

Nutrition:

133 Calories

8.85g Fat

10g Protein

Apple Salad

Preparation Time: 15 minutes

Cooking Time: 5 minutes

Servings: 4

Ingredients:

- 1 medium apple
- 2 oz pecans
- 16 oz broccoli florets
- 1 green onion
- 2 tsp poppy seeds
- Salt and ground black pepper to taste
- ¼ cup sour cream
- ¼ cup mayonnaise
- ½ tsp lemon juice
- 1 tsp apple cider vinegar

Directions:

1. Core and grate apple. Chop pecans and broccoli florets. Dice green onion. In bowl, combine broccoli, apple, pecans, and green onion. Stir well.

2. Sprinkle with poppy seeds, black pepper and salt, stir carefully. In another bowl, whisk sour cream, mayonnaise, lemon juice and vinegar.

3. Add this mixture to salad and toss to coat. Serve.

Nutrition:

249 Calories

22.9g Fat

4.8g Protein

Bok Choy Salad

Preparation Time: 20 minutes

Cooking Time: 10 minutes

Servings: 6

Ingredients:

- 10 oz bok choy, chopped roughly
- 2 tbsp coconut oil
- 4 tbsp chicken stock
- 1 tsp basil
- 1 tsp ground black pepper
- 1 white onion, peeled and sliced
- ¼ cup white mushrooms, marinated and chopped
- 1 lb. tofu, chopped
- 1 tsp oregano
- 1 tsp almond milk

Directions:

1. Heat up pan on medium heat. Add bok choy, 1 tablespoon of oil and chicken stock.
2. Season with basil and black pepper. Add onion and close lid.
3. Simmer vegetables for 5-6 minutes, stirring constantly. Transfer vegetables to bowl and

add mushrooms. Pour 1 tablespoon of oil in pan and heat it up again.

4. Add chopped tofu and cook for 2 minutes. Transfer tofu to bowl with vegetables and sprinkle with oregano. Pour in almond milk and toss to coat.

5. Serve salad.

Nutrition:

130 Calories

4.67g Carbs

11g Fat

6.9g Protein

Halloumi Salad

Preparation Time: 15 minutes

Cooking Time: 12 minutes

Servings: 2

Ingredients:

- 3 oz halloumi cheese, sliced
- 1 cucumber, sliced
- ½ cup baby arugula
- 5 cherry tomatoes, halved
- 1 oz walnuts, chopped
- Salt and ground black pepper to taste
- ½ tsp olive oil
- ¼ tsp balsamic vinegar

Directions:

1. Preheat grill on medium high heat. Put halloumi cheese in grill and cook for 5 minutes per side.
2. In mixing bowl, combine cucumber, arugula, tomatoes, and walnuts. Place halloumi pieces on top.
3. Sprinkle with black pepper and salt. Drizzle oil and balsamic vinegar, toss to coat.
4. Serve.

Nutrition:

448 Calories

3.98g Carbs

42.8g Fat

22.3g Protein

Smoked Salmon Salad

Preparation Time: 17 minutes

Cooking Time: 10 minutes

Servings: 4

Ingredients:

- 8 oz smoked salmon, sliced into thin pieces
- 2 oz pecans, crushed
- 3 medium tomatoes, chopped
- ½ cup lettuce, chopped
- 1 cucumber, diced
- 1/3 cup cream cheese
- 1/3 cup coconut milk
- ½ tsp oregano
- 1 tbsp lemon juice, chopped
- ½ tsp basil
- 1 tsp salt

Directions:

1. In medium bowl, combine salmon with pecans and stir. Add tomatoes, lettuce and cucumber, stir well.

2. In another bowl, mix together cream cheese, coconut milk, oregano, lemon juice, basil and salt. Stir mixture until get homogenous mass. Serve salmon salad with cream cheese sauce.

Nutrition:

211 Calories

15.9g Fat

9.95g Protein

Tuna Salad

Preparation Time: 18 minutes

Cooking Time: 10 minutes

Servings: 4

Ingredients:

- 1 can tuna
- 4 eggs, boiled, peeled and chopped
- 1 oz olives, pitted and sliced
- 1/3 cup cheese cream
- ½ cup almond milk
- ½ tsp ground black pepper
- ½ tsp kosher salt
- 1 tbsp garlic, minced

Directions:

1. In medium bowl, mash tuna with fork. Add chopped eggs and stir. Add sliced olives and stir.

2. In another bowl, whisk together cheese cream and almond milk. Add black pepper, salt and garlic, stir carefully. Add cheese mixture to tuna mixture and mix up. Serve.

Nutrition:

182 Calories

11.9g Fat

12.88g Protein

Caprese Salad

Preparation Time: 7 minutes

Cooking Time: 10 minutes

Servings: 2

Ingredients:

- 8 oz mozzarella cheese
- 1 medium tomato
- 4 basil leaves
- Salt and ground black pepper to taste
- 3 tsp balsamic vinegar
- 1 tbsp olive oil

Directions:

1. Slice mozzarella cheese and tomato. Torn basil leaves. Alternate tomato and mozzarella slices on 2 plates. Season with pepper and salt. Drizzle vinegar and olive oil. Sprinkle with the basil leaves.
2. Serve.

Nutrition:

148 Calories

5.9g Carbs

11.8g Fat

8.95g Protein

Warm Bacon Salad

Preparation Time: 16 minutes

Cooking Time: 18 minutes

Servings: 5

Ingredients:

- 16 oz bacon strips, chopped
- 1 tsp cilantro
- 1 tsp ground ginger
- 1 tsp kosher salt
- 2 tbsp butter
- 3 boiled eggs, peeled and chopped
- 2 tomatoes, diced
- 1 oz spinach, chopped
- 4 oz Cheddar cheese, grated
- 1 tsp almond milk
- 7 oz eggplant, peeled and diced

Directions:

1. In medium bowl, combine bacon, cilantro, ginger and salt. Heat up pan over medium heat and melt 1 tablespoon of butter. Put bacon in pan and cook for 5 minutes. Transfer bacon to plate.
2. Meanwhile, in bowl, mix together chopped eggs, tomatoes and spinach. Sprinkle with

cheese and add almond milk. Heat up pan again over medium heat and melt remaining 1 tablespoon of butter.

3. Add diced eggplants and fry for 8 minutes, stirring occasionally. Then add bacon and roasted eggplants to salad. Season with salt and stir gently. Serve.

Nutrition:

159 Calories

4.22g Carbs

13g Fat

8.75g Protein

Cauliflower Side Salad

Preparation Time: 14 minutes

Cooking Time: 7 minutes

Servings: 8

Ingredients:

- 21 oz cauliflower
- 1 tbsp water
- 4 boiled eggs, peeled and chopped
- 1 cup onion, chopped
- 1 cup celery, chopped
- 1 cup mayonnaise
- Salt and ground black pepper to taste
- 2 tbsp cider vinegar
- 1 tsp sucralose

Directions:

1. Divide cauliflower into florets and put them in heatproof bowl. Add water and place in microwave, cook for 5 minutes. Transfer to serving bowl.
2. Add eggs, onions, and celery. Stir gently. In another bowl, whisk together mayonnaise, black pepper, salt, vinegar and sucralose. Add this sauce to salad and toss to coat. Serve.

Nutrition:

209 Calories

2.9g Carbs

19.7g Fat

3.97g Protein

Ketogenic Tricolor Salad

Preparation Time: 12 minutes

Cooking Time: 8 minutes

Servings: 5

Ingredients:

- 5 oz mozzarella cheese
- 1 tsp oregano
- 1 tsp minced garlic
- 1 tsp basil
- 1 tbsp coconut oil
- 1 tsp lemon juice
- 2 medium tomatoes, sliced
- 7 oz avocado, pitted and sliced
- 8 olives, pitted and sliced

Directions:

1. Cut mozzarella cheese balls into halves. In medium bowl, mix together oregano, garlic, basil, coconut oil and lemon juice.
2. On serving plate place sliced tomato, then place sliced avocado and olives. Put mozzarella pieces on top. Drizzle coconut sauce over salad and serve.

Nutrition:

239 Calories

7.9g Carbs

20.1g Fat

11.77g Protein

Low Carb Chicken Salad with Chimichurri Sauce

Preparation Time: 10 minutes

Cooking Time: 15 minutes

Serving: 5

Ingredients:

- 250 grams of various lettuce leaves
- 2 medium chicken breasts
- 2 medium avocados
- ¼ cup olive oil
- 3 tablespoons red wine vinegar
- ¼ cup parsley
- 1 tablespoon oregano
- 1 teaspoon chili pepper
- 1 teaspoon garlic

Directions:

1. Preheat the non-stick skillet. Place the lettuce and diced avocado in a salad bowl. Cook the chicken breasts, fry them until white. Let the chicken cool.
2. In a small bowl, combine olive oil, vinegar, parsley, oregano, garlic, and chili. Cut the chicken breast into cubes. Add the chopped chicken fillet to the salad and season with the classic chimichurri sauce.

3. Garnish the salad with additional chimichurri sauce and serve.

Nutrition:

285.94 calories

21.24 g fat

17.24 g protein.

Potluck Lamb Salad

Preparation Time: 20 minutes

Cooking Time: 10 minutes

Servings: 4

Ingredients:

- 2 tbsp. olive oil, divided
- 12 oz. grass-fed lamb leg steaks
- 6½ oz. halloumi cheese
- 2 jarred roasted red bell peppers
- 2 cucumbers, cut into thin ribbons
- 3 C. fresh baby spinach
- 2 tbsp. balsamic vinegar

Directions:

1. In a skillet, heat 1 tbsp. of the oil over medium-high heat and cook the lamb steaks for about 4-5 minutes per side or until desired doneness. Transfer the lamb steaks onto a cutting board for about 5 minutes. Then cut the lamb steaks into thin slices. In the same skillet, add haloumi and cook for about 1-2 minutes per side or until golden.

2. In a salad bowl, add the lamb, haloumi, bell pepper, cucumber, salad leaves, vinegar, and remaining oil and toss to combine.

3. Serve immediately.

Nutrition:

420 Calories

35.4g Protein

1.3g Fiber

Spring Supper Salad

Preparation Time: 15 minutes

Cooking Time: 5 minutes

Servings: 5

Ingredients:

For Salad:

- 1 lb. fresh asparagus
- ½ lb. smoked salmon
- 2 heads red leaf lettuce
- ¼ C. pecans

For Dressing:

- ¼ C. olive oil
- 2 tbsp. fresh lemon juice
- 1 tsp. Dijon mustard

Directions:

1. In a pan of boiling water, add the asparagus and cook for about 5 minutes. Drain the asparagus well. In a serving bowl, add the asparagus and remaining salad ingredients and mix. In another bowl, add all the dressing ingredients and beat until well combined. Place the dressing over salad and gently, toss to coat well. Serve immediately.

Nutrition:

223 Calories

8.5g Carbohydrates

3.5g Fiber

Chicken-of-Sea Salad

Preparation Time: 15 minutes

Cooking Time: 5 minutes

Servings: 6

Ingredients:

- 2 (6-oz.) cans olive oil-packed tuna
- 2 (6-oz.) cans water packed tuna
- ¾ C. mayonnaise
- 2 celery stalks
- ¼ of onion
- 1 tbsp. fresh lime juice
- 2 tbsp. mustard
- 6 C. fresh baby arugula

Directions:

1. In a large bowl, add all the ingredients except arugula and gently stir to combine. Divide arugula onto serving plates and top with tuna mixture. Serve immediately.

Nutrition:

325 Calories

27.4g Protein

1.1g Fiber

Ketogenic Kohlrabi Salad

Preparation Time: 10 minutes

Cooking Time: 0 minute

Servings: 2

Ingredients:

- 450g kohlrabi
- 225 ml plain mayonnaise

Directions:

1. Clean the kohlrabi. Cut out any tough parts of the cabbage. Mix mayonnaise to the cabbage. Season the kohlrabi salad.

Nutrition:

4g Fiber

41g Fat

405 calories

Fresh Broccoli Salad

with Pancetta

Preparation Time: 10 minutes

Cooking Time: 15 minutes

Servings: 3

Ingredients:

- 150g raw broccoli
- 10 g toasted almonds
- 5g red onion
- 2 pieces of pancetta

Sauce

- 50g mayonnaise
- 10g mustard
- 7g reduced balsamic

Directions:

1. Bake the pancetta for 15 minutes at 160 degrees C. Cut raw broccoli into small pieces, rinse well and dry. Thinly chop the red onion.
2. Mix broccoli, onion, mustard, mayonnaise and balsamic sauce. Add the almonds. Garnish pancetta on top and pour sauce over it.

Nutrition:

301 calories

5g fiber

14g protein

Chicken Salad with Guacamole and Cajun Sauce

Preparation Time: 15 minutes

Cooking Time: 15 minutes

Serving: 2

Ingredients:

- 4 teaspoons sweet paprika powder
- 3 tbsp. dried thyme
- 2 cloves of garlic
- 1 pinch cayenne pepper
- 1 tbsp. olive oil
- 450g chicken breast
- 200g sugar peas
- 4 tomatoes
- 3 tbsp. olive oil
- 1 avocado
- 1 lime juice
- 50g arugula salad

Directions:

1. Prep the Cajun spice mixture. Combine paprika, thyme, garlic, cayenne pepper and olive oil. Cut the chicken into long strips. Sprinkle with the spicy mixture. Marinate for at least 5 minutes. Boil water into a saucepan. Add peas and cook.

2. Portion tomatoes into quarters and remove the core and seeds. Cut the tomatoes into thin strips. Save the pulp for the vinaigrette dressing.

3. Make a French vinaigrette dressing with tomato pulp, 2: 3 volumes of olive oil, and salt and pepper.

4. Peel the avocado; Mix pulp and lime juice. Season then mashed the avocado.

5. Situate skillet over medium heat, fry the chicken in olive oil for 15 minutes. Sprinkle the tomatoes and peas over arugula. Divide the guacamole and chicken strips. Serve the vinaigrette dressing separately.

Nutrition:

18g Fiber

57g Protein

927 calories

Salad with Asparagus, Eggs and Bacon

Preparation Time: 15 minutes

Cooking Time: 5 minutes

Serving: 4

Ingredients:

- 450 g green asparagus
- 75g bacon
- 2 large eggs, boiled
- 2 tbsp. olive oil
- 2 tbsp. red wine vinegar
- 1 tbsp. Dijon mustard
- 1 tbsp. bacon fat
- 1 garlic clove
- 1 pinch salt
- 1 pinch red chili flakes

Directions:

1. Cut the asparagus into 5-centimeter pieces.
2. Boil salted water, add the asparagus and cook for 4 minutes. Remove the asparagus from water and place it in ice bath.
3. Combine oil, vinegar, mustard, bacon grease, garlic, salt, and chili flakes.

4. Sprinkle bacon on top and place in hard-boiled eggs. Season with the dressing. Place the rest of the sauce on the side of the same dish.

Nutrition:

3g Fiber

8g Protein

237 calories

Cauliflower Salad

Preparation Time: 15 minutes

Cooking Time: 25 minutes

Serving: 6

Ingredients:

Cauliflower salad:

- 700 g large cauliflower
- 125 ml water
- 150 g bacon
- 3 stalks of celery
- ½ red onion
- 2 tbsp. onion feathers

Dressing:

- 350 ml mayonnaise
- ¾ tbsp. Dijon mustard
- ¾ tbsp. apple cider vinegar

Directions:

1. Cauliflower salad:
2. Preheat your grill.
3. Cut the cauliflower into slices. Divide and place them on two separate lined sheets. Season.
4. Raise the edges of the foil to cover. Pour 1/4 cup water each over the cauliflower foil sheet. Cover the top with another foil and wrap. Grill

for 20 minutes, keeping the center out of the heat and leaving room for the bacon.

5. Place the bacon slices in a high-sided grill pan. Bake for 15 minutes. Turn them over to the other side 5-7 minutes after starting to bake.
6. Chop the celery stalks, red onion and onion feathers.
7. Remove bacon from grill. Chop.
8. Take out the cauliflower. Let cool. After cooling mix bacon, celery, onion. Save some green onions for decoration.
9. Dressing:
10. Mix mayonnaise, mustard, and apple cider vinegar. Season.
11. Pour the dressing and mix well. Top with bacon and green onions.

Nutrition:

3g Fiber

6g Protein

512 calories

Ketogenic Salad with Chicken, Pesto and Cherry Tomatoes

Preparation Time: 10 minutes

Cooking Time: 20 minutes

Serving: 6

Ingredients:

- 2 tablespoons rosemary
- ½ cup olive oil
- ¼ cups of apple cider vinegar
- ¼ teaspoon garlic paste
- 1 tablespoon mayonnaise
- 600 g chicken fillet
- 6 cups assorted salad greens
- 10 (170 g) cherry tomatoes
- ½ medium avocado
- 30g chopped purple onion
- 2 tablespoons Parmesan cheese

Directions:

1. Finely chop the rosemary.
2. For dressing:
3. Mix oil, vinegar, garlic paste, mayonnaise, and rosemary.
4. Drizzle remaining rosemary over the chicken and season.

5. Preheat a skillet over medium heat, grill the chicken for 20 minutes, and flip over 10 minutes after starting to fry.
6. Let the chicken cool.
7. Mix variety of herbs, cherry tomatoes, chopped onions and avocado.
8. Slice the chicken and place on top. Sprinkle with Parmesan cheese.

Nutrition:

338 calories

24.7g fat

23.8g protein

Roasted Salmon Salad

with Sesame Oil

Preparation Time: 10 minutes

Cooking Time: 20 minutes

Serving: 6

Ingredients

Salad

- 1 medium lettuce
- 1 medium red pepper
- 1 medium yellow pepper
- 2 large pieces salmon fillet
- 4 tablespoons olive oil
- 1 teaspoon sesame oil
- 2 tablespoons of coconut amino acids
- ¼ cup green onions

Dressing

- 4 tablespoons olive oil
- 1 teaspoon sesame oil
- 5 tablespoons of coconut amino acids

Directions:

1. Heat ¾ olive oil over medium heat. Mix sesame oil, coconut oil, and liquid amino acids. Chop the salmon. Cook salmon slices for 7 minutes.

2. Turnover, continue cooking for another 5 minutes. Put the lettuce and bell peppers in bowl.

3. Once done, place salmon on top of the lettuce and pepper leaves, add the dressing, stir the salad and enjoy!

Nutrition:

383 calories

27.14g fat

24.3g protein.

Diet Salad with

Bacon and Broccoli

Preparation Time: 15 minutes

Cooking Time: 10 minutes

Servings: 6

Ingredients:

- 340 g broccoli cabbage
- 6 slices fried bacon
- 1/2 medium red onion
- 5 tablespoons mayonnaise
- 1 teaspoon erythritol
- 1 tablespoon apple cider vinegar

Directions:

1. Fry the bacon in a preheated skillet. Mix broccoli and onions. Whisk the mayonnaise, erythritol, and apple cider vinegar together.
2. Slice bacon, then add it to the broccoli. Stir well and pour into the broccoli bowl. Stir again, spreading the dressing evenly.

Nutrition:

155.5 calories

12.92g fat

5.4g protein.

Cobb Ketogenic Salad with Chicken and Vinaigrette Dressing

Preparation Time: 10 minutes

Cooking Time: 25 minutes

Servings: 6

Ingredients:

Salad

- 1 package "spring mix"
- 6 slices of bacon
- 2 small cooked chicken breasts
- 3 large hard-boiled eggs
- 1 medium avocado
- 1/3 cups green onions
- ½ cup blue cheese
- 1 cup cherry tomatoes

Vinaigrette dressing

- 1/3 cup olive oil
- 0.25 cups wine vinegar
- 1/2 tablespoon Dijon mustard
- ½ tablespoon sugar substitute

Directions:

1. Mix all salad ingredients. Blend the vinaigrette ingredients until completely dissolved.
2. Season the salad.

Nutrition:

344.12 calories

26.27 g fat

21.12 g protein.

Ketogenic Salad with Canned Tuna and Pesto Sauce

Preparation Time: 10 minutes

Cooking Time: 0 minute

Serving: 1

Ingredients:

Dressing

- 1 tablespoon olive oil
- ½ tbsp. tablespoons apple cider vinegar

Salad

- 4 large iceberg lettuce leaves
- 1 small tomato
- ½ small cucumber
- ¼ medium avocado

Tuna

- 1 can of canned tuna in oil
- tablespoons mayonnaise
- 1 tablespoon pesto sauce
- 2 teaspoons lemon juice

Directions:

1. Incorporate olive oil, apple cider vinegar, and some salt and pepper. Prep the ingredients for the salad by shredding the lettuce leaves. Slice

the tomatoes, cucumber, and avocado then arrange on top of the salad.

2. Toss the tuna, mayonnaise, yogurt, pesto, lemon juice, and some salt. Add the tuna mix to the top of the salad, then drizzle the dressing over the top.

Nutrition:

604.8 calories

46.5 g fat

34.5 g protein

Ketogenic Peanut Butter Bars

Preparation Time: 5 minutes

Cooking Time: 15 minutes

Serving: 10

Ingredients:

- Half a cup of coconut flour
- Two cups of peanut butter that is smooth
- Half cup of sweetener that is sticky

Directions:

1. Place a parchment paper in a square pan and line it with it
2. Put all the ingredients into a big mixing bowl and mix until it is fully combined
3. Pour the batter into the already lined baking pan and refrigerate it till it is firm.
4. When it is firm, cut it into 20 bars and serve.

Nutrition:

112 calories

8g Fat

4g Carbohydrates

4g Protein

3g Fiber

Ketogenic Chocolate Crunch Bars

Preparation Time: 5 minutes

Cooking Time: 10 minutes

Serving: 10

Ingredients:

- One and a half cup of chocolate chips (of choice)
- One cup of almond butter (or any seed/nut butter of choice)
- A quarter cup of coconut oil
- Half cup of sweetener that is sticky
- Three cups of almond nuts or cashew nuts (or any other nuts you desire)

Directions:

1. Get a big baking dish and line it with parchment paper.
2. Get a bowl that is microwave friendly and mix the chocolate chips, the coconut oil, the almond butter and the sweetener and melt them till they combine.
3. Then add the almond nut or the cashew nut or your desired nuts and combine the mixture well by mixing it.

4. Pour the mixture into the already lined baking dish and let it spread.
5. Refrigerate the mixture till it is firm. When it is firm, cut it into 20 bars and serve.

Nutrition:

155 calories

12g Fat

4g Carbohydrate

7g Protein

2g Fiber

Ketogenic Coconut Chocolate Bars

Preparation Time: 5 minutes

Cooking Time: 10 minutes

Serving: 10

Ingredients:

- Two cups of any type of chocolate chips desired
- One cup of coconut oil that is melted
- Three cups of coconut flakes that is shredded
- A quarter cup of sweetener

Directions:

1. Use a parchment paper to line the inside of a big baking pan. Get a big mixing bowl and put all of the ingredients. Mix the mixture to let it be well combined
2. Pour the batter (the mixture) in the already lined with parchment paper pan. Use your hands to press it firmly. Wet your hands to press it.
3. Refrigerate to make it firm. When it is firm, remove from the refrigerator and cut it into 20 bars and put it back in the refrigerator.
4. Melt the chocolate chips and dip each of the coconut bars into the melted chocolate. Refrigerate again and serve.

Nutrition:

106 Calories

11g Total fat

3g Total carbohydrate

2g Protein

Ketogenic Lemon Bars

Preparation Time: 30 minutes

Cooking Time: 15 minutes

Serving: 4

Ingredients:

- Three lemons
- One and a half cup of almond flour
- Half a cup of butter
- One cup of powdered sweetener

Directions:

1. Get a baking dish and line it with parchment paper. Mix a cup of the almond flour, a quarter of the sweetener, the butter and a pinch of salt together in a medium mixing bowl. Pour this mixture into the baking dish that is already lined with parchment paper and bake for about 20 minutes. Remove and let it cool down.

2. Zest one of the lemons in a medium bowl and juice the three lemons. Put the eggs and the rest of the sweetener, the rest of the almond flour and add a pinch of salt. Mix together to make the filling.

3. This filling can now be poured into the baked crust and bake for 15 minutes. Remove and

serve with slices of lemon. Also sprinkle sweetener on it.

Nutrition:

193 calories

19 g Fat

4g Protein

3g Carbohydrates

Chocolate Chip Pumpkin Protein Bar

Preparation Time: 5 minutes

Cooking Time: 10 minutes

Serving: 4

Ingredients:

- Two table spoons of chocolate chips that is sugar free
- Half a cup of coconut flour
- Three table spoons of protein powder
- Half a cup of pumpkin puree
- One table spoon of pumpkin pie spice
- Three table spoons of butter powder
- A pinch of salt
- Half cup of almond milk that is unsweetened
- Two table spoons of powdered sweetener

Directions:

1. Get a medium baking pan and line it with parchment paper Get a medium mixing bowl; add the butter powder flour, the protein powder, a pinch of salt, the coconut flour, the powdered sweetener and the pumpkin pie spice. Mix together until they are well combined.

2. Add the pumpkin puree and the almond milk and stir well until they have combined well. Also add the chocolate chips and stir.

3. Pour the mixture into the baking pan and make it firm by pressing it down. Refrigerate for some minutes and slice in to bars, then serve.

Nutrition:

89.1 Calories

2.7g Fat

7.1g Protein

5.7g Carbohydrate

Ketogenic Flourless Chocolate Cake

Preparation Time: 10 minutes

Cooking Time: 30 minutes

Serving: 4

Ingredients:

- One and a half cup of cocoa powder
- Two table spoons of baking powder
- Two and a half spoons of Dutch cocoa
- One and a half cup of milk (use a plant-based milk like coconut milk, almond milk or other plant-based milk of choice for the vegan version of the Ketogenic flourless chocolate cake)
- One and a half table spoon of flavor of choice
- One cup of sugar (coconut sugar or date sugar of half of a cup of erythritol for the gluten free version)

Directions:

1. First of all, heat the oven to about 350F Get a baking pan and line it with the parchment paper
2. In a big mixing bowl, mix all the dry ingredients (the cocoa powder, the Dutch cocoa, the baking powder, the coconut sugar or the date sugar Use a mixer to whisk the eggs. Do this till the size has doubled and till it is frothy.

3. In another small mixing bowl, mix the wet ingredients (the milk and the flavor) gently add the mixed wet ingredients to the mixed dry ingredients and stir.

4. Pour the mixture into the already lined baking pan with parchment paper. Bake for about 30 minutes. Remove from baking pan and serve

Nutrition:

130 Calories

9g Total Fat

0.9g Saturated Fat

175mg Sodium

Brownie Cheese Cake

Preparation Time: 15 minutes

Cooking Time: 30 minutes

Serving: 4

Ingredients:

- Almond flour or coconut flour (that is finely ground)
- Butter (soft
- Erythritol (the powdered form)
- Cocoa powder: (Dutch baking cocoa powder)
- Vanilla extract (that is free of sugar)
- Cream cheese (the full fat type)
- Some chocolate bars (to be grated)

Directions:

1. For the brownie layer
2. Mix the Dutch baking cocoa powder and the vanilla extract in a mixing bowl until it has combined well add the soft butter and mix well. (be sure to make the butter mix well in the mixture to form a paste)
3. Pour the mixture (the brownie layer) halfway into an appropriate silicon mold of the desired size (be sure to fill it halfway to allow for the cheese layer to also be poured in it)

4. The brownie layer can be stored in a fridge pending the time the cheesecake layer would be ready.
5. For the cheese cake layer
6. Add the rest of the butter, the almond flour or coconut flour, the rest of the vanilla essence into a mixing bowl and mix till it is very smooth.
7. When it is very smooth, pour the mixture into the cooled half-filled silicon mold till it is filled up. Freeze in a freezer for about 2 hours or till it is hard enough.
8. Remove the already made brownie cheesecake from the silicon mold carefully and serve.

Nutrition:

231 Calories

16.4g Total Fat

182mg Sodium

22.1g Total Carbohydrate

Peanut Butter Molten

Lava Cake

Preparation Time: 25 minutes

Cooking Time: 15 minutes

Servings: 4

Ingredients:

- 2 very big eggs and their yolks
- A cup of peanut butter
- Chocolate sauce (that is low carb)
- Six full table spoons of almond flour
- one full table spoons of vanilla essence
- two table spoons of coconut oil
- seven tablespoons of sweetener (powered form)
- a spoon of butter to grease the baking pan

Directions:

1. Heat the oven to about 370F. Use the butter to grease the baking pan very well so that the cake would remove smoothly without any dent.
2. Put the coconut oil and peanut butter into a bowl that is microwave safe and stir. Heat them for a little while to get it melted. When the mixture is already melted, stir it well till it mixes together and is smooth.

3. Add the powdered sweetener into the melted mixture and whisk it. Also add the almond flour, the vanilla essence, the eggs and their yolks. Shake and mix together the mixture until it is very smooth.

4. Fill the baking pan with the barter and bake for about 15 minutes. Once done, remove the cake from the pan using a knife to loosen the cake from the baking pan.

5. Place on a serving plate and drizzle it with the chocolate sauce (that is low in carbohydrate) Follow this process for the four cakes

Nutrition:

387 Calories

35.02g Total Fat

10.44g Protein

6.41g Carbohydrate

1.13g Fiber

www.ingramcontent.com/pod-product-compliance
Lightning Source LLC
Chambersburg PA
CBHW050744030426
42336CB00012B/1656

* 9 7 8 1 8 0 3 4 2 2 7 5 6 *